Ketogenic Diet for Beginners

Start Your Keto Diet, Easy Recipes and Change Your Life

Table of Contents

Introduction

I want to thank you and congratulate you for purchasing this book, *"Ketogenic Diet for Beginners: Start Your Keto Diet, Easy Recipes and Change Your Life"*.

This book is not just a book for beginners wanting to know more about ketogenic but it also provides a full day meals recipe that you can get started on immediately.

The book is layout with an introduction of what is ketogenic. Before starting any diet, we should be well informed of the benefits ketogenic has for our body. A full week's meal plan is laid out for you, including one of the full day's meals recipe.

Thanks again for purchasing this book and I hope you enjoy it!

Part I – What is Ketogenic Diet?

I have been a health advocate for years. It is truly a life-changing experience for anyone who takes fitness seriously. Your confidence blooms, relationships strengthen and your life improves. Two common ways are through diet or exercise. Here we'll go over the diet part by introducing to you the Ketogenic Diet.

There are numerous diets you can search up on Google that are made to give you different results for your ideal body. But, among the various you may read, today we will be discussing the all glorious, low-carb, high-fat diet known as the Ketogenic Diet.

Ketogenic? What?

For all the Keto-Beginners out there, the word '*Ketogenic*' may be a first for you, but do not worry, for this will be explained further. The word comes from Keto, which was coined when your body reduces carbs into a form of metabolism called Ketosis. At this state, your body becomes a superhero and is able to burn fat for energy in an incredibly efficient manner.

Basically, as mentioned earlier on, it is a very low-carb, high-fat diet that lowers blood sugar and insulin levels that will be able to shift your metabolism away from carbohydrates and turn towards a lot of fat and ketones.

With every diet, comes great benefits and it is no more different with the Ketogenic diet. You can expect that this diet will provide massive reductions in your blood sugar and insulin levels and you know what that means? Well, in the long run, it will be great in fighting against diabetes, cancer, epilepsy and even Alzheimer's disease. Its overall benefits are great for your metabolism (*making you burn fat for energy swift and easy*), neurologically (*yes it does help in recovering brain injuries*) and insulin-related diseases (*diabetes, of course*)

So you may, if not already, want to consider looking into this diet for a healthier future for your mind and body.

Now, a perk that some people may be looking for is: Does this diet make me lose weight? You're in luck, because yes, yes it does! In fact, you may believe it or not, but this Ketogenic diet is far more superior than your typically recommended low-fat diets that definitely make you lose weight, but at the cost of your health. You can even throw away that calorie counter because the diet is actually quite filling that you lose the weight without having to keep track.

Imagine how much more time you would get in your day when you don't need to just constantly be counting on your calories!

The bottom line is that this diet will definitely make you lose more weight than your standard low-fat diet, and you don't have to starve to do it.

To get an idea of the food you are allowed to eat, there is:

- Meats – *such as red meat like steaks, ham, sausages, bacon, chicken, and turkey*
- Fatty Fishes – *delicious salmon is included along with trout, tuna, and mackerel*
- Eggs – *suggest the pastured eggs*
- Butter and Creams – *grass-fed if possible*
- Cheese – *make sure it's unprocessed*
- Nuts and Seeds – *any and all are fine*
- Healthy Oils – *these would only include extra virgin olive oil, coconut, and avocado*
- Avocados – *always great to get healthy fats*
- Low-Carb Veggies – *this just is, most of your typical green veggies*

- Condiments – *herbs and spices! Make your meals tasty!*

Now that the basic idea is out of the way, we can get into the delicious details of some of the great meal plans that you can prepare with this diet!

Just to help you out on how your week is going to be like, I prepared a simple plan to get you started:

Monday

- Breakfast Meal: some crispy bacon and eggs with a side of tomato
- Lunch Meal: chicken salad dressed with olive oil and garnished with feta cheese
- Dinner Meal: pan-fried salmon with a side of asparagus cooked in butter.

Tuesday

- Breakfast Meal: omelet filled with egg, tomato, basil and goat cheese
- Lunch Meal: Stevia milkshake blended with almond milk, peanut butter, cocoa powder (*Stevia* is a natural sweetener that has been proven to provide a lot of health benefits)
- Dinner Meal: meatballs showered with cheddar cheese and a side of vegetables

Wednesday

- Breakfast Meal: Ketogenic Milkshake (*There will be instructions as to how to make this in the next section*)
- Lunch Meal: shrimp salad dressed in olive oil with avocado

- Dinner Meal: pork chops with a side of salad, broccoli, and parmesan cheese

Thursday

- Breakfast Meal: omelet filled with avocado, salsa, peppers, onion and some spices (*Whatever spice that fill your fancy*)
- Lunch Meal: guacamole and salsa dip with nuts and celery sticks
- Dinner Meal: chicken stuffed pesto and cream cheese with a side of vegetables

Friday

- Breakfast Meal: 3-cheese omelet cooked with or a side of tomatoes
- Lunch Meal: some of that leftover chicken you cooked on Thursday (*Make sure to cook a lot!*)
- Dinner Meal: steak with a side of egg, mushrooms and salad

Alternative Friday

- Breakfast Meal: milkshake made with sugar-free yoghurt, peanut butter, cocoa powder, and stevia
- Lunch: beef stir fry cooked in coconut oil with a side of vegetables
- Dinner Meal: bun-less burger with some bacon, egg and sprinkled with cheese (*Or otherwise, known as just burger steak*)

Saturday

- Breakfast Meal: ham and cheese omelet with a side of vegetables
- Lunch Meal: ham and cheese slices with a side of nuts

- Dinner Meal: white fish cooked with coconut oil and a side of egg and spinach

Sunday

- Breakfast Meal: fried eggs with eggs and a side of mushroom
- Lunch Meal: burger dressed with salsa, cheese, and guacamole
- Dinner Meal: steak with eggs and a side of salad

Try to keep in mind to rotate the meat with the side of vegetables, as this is the main concept of the diet. Basically, if you haven't noticed from the meal plan set out that you are still able to eat a wide variety of foods with some nutritious value with this sort of diet.

In order to help you out even more! Here are some more recipes you can try to cook out in your very own home.

Part II – How to Start a Diet

There are many diets that are effective out there and chances are you have heard of more than one type of diet. Ketogenic Diet is just one of many effective diets out there. But when you encounter or planning to start a diet, you may be wondering, "How do I start?". Generally, the perception of starting a diet would involve following a meal plan; what to eat and what not to eat. And that could be just it but it is not. You can discover that further in the following chapters.

The first step of starting a diet can be a challenge for some as they may fall out from schedule half way through or even in the first week of dieting. Have you ever experience starting a diet only to find that it is "Day 3" and you are struggling to continue? If so, you have been overwhelmed. Starting on the right foot is what will get you going in a diet. How do you start a diet?

It's all in the Mind

It really does start with the mind. This concept is nothing new. To start a diet, you got to ask yourself, "Are you ready?". Are you ready to take on a change in your life, especially improving your health? Many fail because they deep dive into a total change that the self cannot take. When getting yourself prepared, understand where you are at and where you want to go in the diet journey. If your mind is not ready, your body is not too. But do not take too long preparing your mind. In the effort to improve your health, you got to challenge yourself. I would suggest asking yourself,

- Do you want to improve your health?
- Can you start step by step or leap by leap?
- So, are you ready?

Once you have the answers in place, take your next step.

What fits?

What fits you? There are many diet out there that works but it varies to what the schedule is like, the meal plans, the cost, the duration of the diet or even availability of the food. Some diet have a list food that may not be available in your area. Even though you may figure out substitutes, but wouldn't it be nice to follow a diet that all the way?

Do some research on which diet fits you best. There may also be diets whereby you are allergic or cannot take certain food in the meal plans. Besides that, if a diet requires strenuous routine that your body is, medically, not up for it, avoid that. Choose a diet that suits you.

Step-by-Step

Set out to take your diet by storm but like all storms, it gradually builds. Take your diet one step at a time. All great diet have plans set out for you and there is a reason for that; Rome wasn't built in a day. Diet takes time and so does your body in its change journey. If you rush and hope to see results instantly, you may be setting yourself up for failure. Set yourself up for success. You will definitely be a storm to be reckoned with at the end of your diet (or even half way through your diet).

Enlist a Buddy

It is essential that you have support in your journey. A buddy is one of that support, whether it is your family members or friends. Having a buddy, especially if your buddy is going through the same diet program as you, will be a source of encouragement if the going gets tough.

Set Realistic Goals

Starting a diet program is great but without an end in mind, you may be going through the diet without realizing what you want out of it. What do you hope to achieve in the diet? When do you want to see changes? Can you achieve X goal by X date?

Setting goals that are realistic will get you to where you want to go. Avoid setting goals that are not realistic; losing XX kg (double digit) in one week. That may sound possible for some hardcore enthusiast but it may not be realistic for many. When you set unrealistic goals, you may fall trap into getting demotivated when you do not achieve them. Additionally, you may set small realistic goals that will act as your milestone. That way, you will be able to track your progress.

Track Your Progress

Tracking your progress helps to know where you are at in your journey. It is also a way to know whether you are achieving the realistic goals you have set. In order to track your progress, you will need a tool to track it. In most cases, a journal is used. However, you are not restricted to a journal. You may track your progress with a smartphone (app). A benefit for having a smartphone is you are bringing your progress with you every day (since you would be bringing your phone around with you). In some apps, you are able to key in your measurements, count calories and even take photo of how fabulous you are progressing.

Wicked Playlist

Most diet programs have exercise incorporated. Chances are, you may not be exercising without music. Set up a playlist for your exercise time. It will get you pumping and motivated to continue on. Besides adding music to your playlist, add in some motivational tracks too. It will be beneficial both mentally and physically to have a great combination of music (to pump you up) and motivation (build your knowledge).

Part III – Delicious Recipes for Fat Loss

One of the keys to success in the world of dieting is to not get bored with what you are eating. A good variety and good tasting foods are a needed for staying on a diet for as long as possible. Thankfully, we have recipes here that will get your fat burning and taste great. Let's start with the first meal of the day.

Breakfast Meal: Ketogenic White Pizza Frittata

Frittatas are great. A versatile breakfast meal, they are easy to prepare, easy to cook, easy to eat when you're in a rush in the morning and can be microwaved, reheated or even eaten just plain cold! All depends on your preferences. This dish is filled with fat from all the cheeses yet only 2g of carbs, this is going to make our body just burn all that fat from the cheese off.

For the recipe mentioned below, the cooking pan used is a cast iron skillet. But if you don't have one it can be just as easily prepared in a glass baking dish, however, if you do use that you may want to consider keeping it in the oven for just a bit longer.

Serving(s): 8

You will need:

- 12 Large Eggs
- 9 ounce Frozen Spinach
- 1 ounce Pepperoni
- 5 ounce Mozzarella Cheese
- 1 teaspoon Garlic – Minced
- ½ cup of Fresh Ricotta Cheese
- ½ cup of Parmesan Cheese
- 4 tablespoon Olive Oil

- ¼ teaspoon Nutmeg
- Salt depending on your taste

What to do:

1. Microwave the frozen spinach until it has been defrosted, this could take around 4 -5 minutes and then drain as much of the water as you can and set it aside.
2. The oven is then should be pre-heated at 375 Fahrenheit while you mix the eggs, olive oil, and spices into a bowl and whisked until all ingredients are mixed together.
3. Once mixed, place the ricotta cheese, Parmesan cheese and squeezed spinach (*Break apart the spinach when placing into the mixing bowl*) and mix.
4. Pour the mixture into your cast iron skillet and sprinkle all that good mozzarella cheese on the top and place some pepperonis along with it.
5. Bake it for 30 minutes or until the center has been cooked. (*If you have the glass container inside the cast iron skillet then it would cook for about 40 – 45 minutes instead*)
6. Take it out of the oven, slice it up and get ready to enjoy some good Ketogenic-style Frittata

Nutritional Value per Serving:

- 298 Calories
- 23.8 grams of Fats
- 2.1 grams of Carbs
- 19.4 grams of Protein

Spinach

It is no secret that leafy greens are good for you and it shouldn't be surprising that spinach (Which was the leafy greens that Popeye used to make himself big and strong) has numerous amounts of health benefits that will help your body fight against countless diseases, some of these benefits are:

- Protect yourself against inflammatory problems
- Oxidative stress-related problems
- Cardiovascular problems
- Bone problems
- Helps fight against cancer

Nutmeg

This popular spice has made its way on top of the list of providing great benefits and has a long list of associated health benefits. Apart from being greatly beneficial, it is also great to add on your dish for a punch of flavor. Some of the benefits include:

- Relieves pain
- Soothes indigestion
- Strengthen cognitive function
- Detoxify the body
- Boost skin health

Bacon and eggs is a classic meal and it is available at almost every breakfast menu. However, to get the right bacon and eggs cook can be frustrating. For a keto diet, bacon and eggs is a great addition to your daily breakfast mix.

Serving(s): 1

You will need:

- 4 slices of bacon
- 3 large eggs
- 3 slices of tomatoes
- 1 tablespoon of butter
- 1/3 cup of heavy cream
- Pinch of salt
- Pinch of black pepper

What to do:

1. Let's start with the bacon. Start by preheating the oven at 350 Fahrenheit.
2. Using a non-stick cookie sheet, spread your bacon on it. Ensure that you don't overlap the bacon.
3. Once your oven is heated, place the bacon into the oven.
4. Set for 10-15 minutes in the oven. Within this time, if you see your bacon looking crispy, you can take them out. Let it cool as you move on to your eggs.
5. Mix the eggs and cream together. Whisk them together lightly.
6. Add butter to the pan over a medium-to-low heat stove.
7. Spread the butter.

8.   As soon as the butter melts and covers the pan, add the egg mixture.
9.   At this point, you are aiming for scrambled eggs, but gently scramble your eggs to ensure your eggs are cooked and the texture is right.
10. When your eggs starts to look runny, you can take them out.
11. Add salt and pepper to taste.
12. Add the eggs, bacon and couple of slice tomatoes. Voila! Enjoy your classic bacon and eggs

Nutritional Value per Serving:

- 690 Calories
- 64 grams of Fats
- 2 grams of Carbs
- 30 grams of Protein

Benefits of this Recipe:

Bacon

For those aiming at low-carb ketogenic diet, bacon is one of the food for you. Although bacon may be perceived as something to avoid, yet it is a must-have in breakfast menu and do have some interesting benefits. Some of the benefits include:

- Low-carb
- Great source for amino acids
- Significant and high-quality protein
- High amounts of HDL (High-Density Lipoprotein) or good cholesterol

Bacon and eggs is a classic meal and it is available at almost every breakfast menu. However, to get the right bacon and eggs cook can be frustrating. For a keto diet, bacon and eggs is a great addition to your daily breakfast mix.

Serving(s): 1-2

You will need:

- 2 tablespoons of unsweetened natural peanut butter
- 2 tablespoons of unsweetened cocoa powder
- 3 tablespoons of whey protein
- 1 cup of unsweetened almond milk
- 2 cups of ice
- 2 tablespoons of heavy whipping cream
- ¼ teaspoon vanilla extract
- ¼ teaspoon stevia powder

What to do:

1. Mix all ingredients into a high-powered blender. Blend until the mixture becomes smooth and creamy

Benefits of this Recipe:

Peanut Butter

Peanut butter is just delicious for kids. There must be childhood memories of licking that peanut butter of a spoon. The mix of peanut butter smoothie has its benefits, such as:

- Prevents cardiovascular disease and coronary heart disease

- Controlling hunger
- Weight management
- Reduce risk of colon cancer

Serving(s): 3-4

You will need:

- 3 tablespoons Olive oil
- 10 eggs
- 5-ounce baby spinach
- 1-pint grape tomatoes, sliced
- 4 scallions, sliced
- 8-ounce feta, crushed
- 1-2 teaspoons salt
- ½ teaspoon fresh and ground pepper
- *Optional*: ¼ cup pitless Greek black olives

What to do:

1. Preheat the oven to 350° F and add oil in a casserole. Keep it in the oven for 5 minutes.
2. Whisk eggs, pepper, and salt together.
3. Add the following in order; tomatoes, scallions, spinach and feta.
4. Take out the casserole from the oven.
5. Transfer mixture to casserole and bake it for 25 to 30 minutes to get puffed and golden in color.

Greek Frittata

Greek frittata is on a calorie count of 636 calories. The benefits of having this meal is that it is low in sugar, calcium level is high. A benefit to the ketogenic diet, fat level for the Greek frittata is high.

Lunch Meal: Bacon, Avocado and Chicken Sandwich

This won't be your typical sandwich since bread is one of the few things you can't eat in a Ketogenic diet. However, if there is a will there is a way because there is Keto Cloud bread that will be a great blend with the Bacon, Avocado, and Chicken. It may sound a little out of the ordinary, but the Keto Cloud bread is actually easy to make and doesn't take too long. If you are planning to keep it around, it can definitely be eaten with anything and saved as batches in your fridge or freezer. The Keto Bread is our main ingredient here which is super low in carbs but high protein and fat.

Serving(s): 2

You will need:

- Electric Mixer

Keto Cloud Bread

- 3 Large Eggs
- 3 ounces of Cream Cheese
- 1/8 teaspoon of Cream Tartar
- ¼ teaspoon Salt
- ½ teaspoon Garlic Powder

The In Between

- 1 tablespoon Mayonnaise
- 1 teaspoon Sriracha
- 2 slices of Bacon
- 3 ounces of Chicken
- 2 slices of Pepper Jack Cheese

- 2 Grape Tomatoes
- ¼ Medium Avocado (this would be about 2 ounces)

What to do:

1. Preheat the oven that is 300° F as you separate the 3 eggs into two separate bowls. One in a bowl with the white yolk and the other with the yellow yolk.
2. Now, add some of that cream of Tartar and salt into your whites. You will need the electric mixer for this and whip the egg whites until it becomes foamy.
3. In the other bowl, combine the 3 ounces of Cubed Cream Cheese with the egg yolks and beat it until it has been combined properly together.
4. Once done, gently fold the egg whites into the yolks. Make sure to do this half at a time.
5. Place parchment paper lined baking sheet on a baking tray and spoon ¼ of the bread batter onto the tray. This should be able to make 6 large Keto cloud bread.
6. With a spatula, press on the Keto Cloud bread batter and try to form into squares. Sprinkle some of that garlic powder and bake it in the oven for about 25 minutes or when you think it looks ready.
7. While the bread bakes, you can now start preparing the chicken and bacon. Just toss the pieces into a pan with some salt and pepper.
8. When creating the sandwich, you can start combining the Sriracha and mayonnaise together and spread it onto the underside of the bread.
9. Place your chicken on the spread
10. Place 2 slices of pepper jack cheese, bacon and some of those grape tomatoes and spread mashed avocado on top.
11. Season to taste and get ready for lunch!

Nutritional Value per Serving:

- 361 Calories
- 28.3 grams of Fat
- 2 grams of Net Carbs
- 22 grams of Protein

Avocado

This fruit is a great gateway to losing weight, improving your skin and lowering life-threatening disease. Specifically speaking:

- Improves cardiovascular health by lessening the risk of coronary heart skin
- Cancer prevention
- Rich in potassium, lowering kidney failure and heart disease
- Protection from wrinkles

Cream of Tartar

One of the main uses for this ingredient is in bakery goods (As is used to make the Keto bread) in order to make it fluffier and lighter. Besides its great use when cooking, it can also be benefited by nutritiously.

- Fight against urinary tract infections
- Help in detoxification for nicotine withdrawals
- Relieves heartburn

Lunch Meal: Guacamole and Salsa Dip

One of the healthiest meal you can prepare easily is the guacamole and salsa dip. To make this healthy, you got to use fresh ingredients.

Serving(s): 4

You will need:

- 4 avocados
- 2 tablespoons jalapeno peppers
- ¼ cup of cilantro
- 2 tablespoons onions
- 2 tomatoes
- 1 garlic clove
- 1 bunch celery
- Salt and black pepper to taste

What to do:

1. Chop the onions, cilantro and jalapeno peppers. Crush your garlic clove. Peeled and diced your tomatoes.
2. Use a fork to mash the avocados.
3. Mix all the ingredients together, except the celery. Celery will be used to dip into your guacamole and salsa dip.

Nutritional Value per Serving:

- 257 Calories
- 22 grams of Fats
- 16 grams of Carbs
- 3.6 grams of Protein

- 10.6 grams of Fiber

Celery

Celery is a great addition for the dip. It can be eaten at its stalks, leaves or, sometimes, its seeds too. In juices, celery is great for balancing out the taste. Not only great for dips, celery has its benefits such as:

- Lowers high cholesterol
- Lowers inflammation
- Reduces bloating
- Reduce high blood pressure

Lunch Meal: Stir-fry Beef and Broccoli

Stir-fry meals are another great option for diet. It is simple to prepare and you can practically stir-fry anything. With this recipe, you can serve it with rice or eat the meal with it.

Serving(s): 4

You will need:

- 4 cups broccoli, chopped (florets)
- 1 lb. boneless round steak
- 3 garlic clove, minced
- 1 small onion
- 1 red bell pepper
- ½ cup water
- 2 tablespoons coconut oil
- 1 teaspoon ground ginger
- ½ tablespoon coconut aminos
- Salt and black pepper to taste
- 1 ½ lb. Brussels sprouts
- Cooking fat

What to do:

1. Use a cast-iron skillet cooked over low-medium heat.
2. Add 2 garlic clove, minced, and cook until its golden.
3. Add Brussels sprouts.
4. Add salt and pepper to taste for about 10-15 minutes. After which, set aside.
5. Use the cast-iron skillet cooked over medium heat to stir-fry the beef for about 6-7 minutes. After which, set the beef aside.
6. Now, time to cook the red bell peppers, broccoli and onions together for about 6 minutes.

7. Add your beef back into the mix.
8. Separately, mix water, ground ginger, remaining garlic, coconut aminos, and salt and pepper to taste. After mixing them together, add it to the beef mix for about 3 minutes.
9. Heat up your Brussels sprouts just right.
10. Once done, add your Brussels sprouts and stir-fry beef together. Voila!

Nutritional Value per Serving:

- 245 Calories
- 5 grams of Fats
- 10 grams of Carbs
- 25 grams of Protein

Benefits of this Recipe:

Broccoli

Whether broccoli is sautéed, stir-fry or just eaten raw, broccoli has its benefits such as:

- Vitamin K for calcium absorption
- Natural detoxification
- Lower heart disease risk
- Lower blood pressure
- Lower cholesterol levels

Dinner Meal: Slow Cooker Keto Chicken Tikka Masala

If you don't know what Tikka Masala is, it is a flavorful curry that would be a great dinner meal. You can choose between eating it on its own and have a side of some great vegetables to up your nutritional value. This recipe will include some cauliflower rice along with the curry.

The amount of condiments that are in Indian cuisine allow for a lot of fat and the chicken proves us with protein. This meal is great for bed because it's high in calories, protein and fat which we can burn in our sleep.

Serving(s): 5

You will need:

- 1 ½ pounds of Chicken Thighs, bone-in and skin-on
- 1 pound of Chicken Thighs, boneless and skinless
- 2 tablespoon of Olive Oil
- 2 teaspoon of Onion Powder
- 3 Cloves of Minced Garlic
- 1 inch of Grated Ginger Root
- 3 tablespoon of Tomato Paste
- 5 teaspoon Garam Masala (*Spice in Tikka Masala*)
- 2 teaspoon of Smoked Paprika
- 4 teaspoon of Kosher Salt
- 10 ounce of Diced Tomatoes
- 1 cup of Heavy Cream
- 1 cup of Coconut Milk (*Carton*)
- Fresh Cilantro (*Chopped for the dressing*)
- 1 teaspoon of Guar Gum (*Powdered Thickener*)

What to do (*Curry*):

1. De-bone the chicken from the bone-in Chicken Thighs and then chop all the chicken pieces into small bite sized pieces. Make sure that the skin is still intact and if you do have the kitchen shears, which will help to cut the chicken.
2. Once done, add some chicken to the slow cooker and grate the ginger over the top.
3. Add the dry spices into the slow cooker and make sure that it has been mixed well.
4. Once done, add the diced tomatoes with the tomato paste into the slow cooker and make sure you mix well.
5. The last ingredient to put into a slow cooker is the ½ cup of coconut milk and mix together thoroughly. Now you will have to cook for 6 hours on low or if you're in a rush then the high for 3 hours
6. Once the slow cooker has done its job, and then you will need to add the leftover coconut milk, heavy cream, and guar gum into the mix. This should thicken the curry and would be served well with the cauliflower rice.

What to do (*Cauliflower Rice*):

1. Sauté Cauliflower rice into a dry pan.
2. Once the cauliflower has been dried out, then add butter, cumin and coriander onto the rice.
3. Add salt and pepper to taste so that the moisture leakage is lowered.

Nutritional Value per Serving:

- 492 Calories
- 41.2 grams of Fat
- 5.8 grams of Carbohydrates
- 26 grams of Protein

Benefits of this Recipe:

Coconut Milk

To clear something up, coconut milk is different from coconut water. Coconut milk is extracted from the coconut milk, which is first skinned and squeezed. Some of the nutritional highlights are as follows:

- Rich in fibre
- Lactose free
- Contains Vitamins C, E, B1, B3, B5 and B6
- Minerals include: Iron, Selenium, Sodium, Calcium, Magnesium and Phosphorous

Ginger

For those of you who may not be very aware that ginger is in fact a great source of nutrition, it is without a doubt a great source of health benefits. Greatly used in numerous recipes and a long history of use for relieving digestive problems, it can beneficial in other ways.

- Relieves nausea, loss of appetite and motion sickness.
- Reduces pain and inflammation
- Improves absorption of nutrients
- Rid of throat and nose congestion

Dinner Meal: French Toast in Crock Pot

Serving(s): 8 – 9

You will need:

- 2 egg whites
- 1 1/2 cups soy or almond milk
- 2 whole eggs
- 1 teaspoon vanilla extract
- 2 tablespoon honey
- 1/2 teaspoon cinnamon powder
- 9 slices whole grain bread

For filling:

- 3 cups apple, finely chopped
- 1 teaspoon lime juice, fresh
- 1/3 cup pecans, raw and diced
- 1/2 teaspoon cinnamon powder
- 3 tablespoon honey

What to do:

1. Take a bowl and add whole eggs, honey, milk, egg whites, vanilla extract and cinnamon powder to mix them well. Grease your slow cooker with the cooking spray. Add all the filling ingredients in a small bowl. Mix well to coat apple pieces and keep them aside.
2. Cut slices of bread into triangular shapes and start with the layer of bread in the bottom of slow cooker. Now add a 1/4th mixture of the filling mixture and add 3 layers of bread. The remaining filling will be added on the top. Pour the mixture of eggs on the bread and cover the slow cooker on high setting for 2.5 hours and

low setting for 4 hours. The bread should soak the liquids. You can use bananas as a substitute of apples.

Nutritional Value per Serving:

- 390 Calories
- 18 grams of Fat
- 32 grams of Carbohydrates
- 23 grams of Protein

Dinner Meal: Beef Noodles

Serving(s): 4

You will need:

- 5 to 6-ounce Cellophane noodles
- 1/3 cup Soy sauce
- 5 tablespoons Sesame oil
- 1 clove minced garlic
- 1/3 cup brown sugar
- 1 1/2 tablespoons apple vinegar
- 12-ounce skirt steak (1/4 inch thick slices)
- 1/4-inch wedges onion
- Kosher salt to taste
- 10 ounces Shiitake mushrooms (remove stems)
- 1 cup shredded carrots
- 6 cups baby spinach

What to do:

1. In the first step, you have to soak noodles in water (warm water) for almost 5 – 10 minutes. Drain water and snip noodle into pieces with kitchen scissors.
2. It is time to take a bowl and mix sesame oil (3 tablespoons), soy sauce, garlic, vinegar and brown sugar. Keep it aside. It is time to put beef to another and add two tablespoons soy sauce mixture. Keep it aside.
3. Take a large cooking pan and heat two teaspoons oil. Add salt and onion in this pan and cook for two minutes. Now, add beef and let it cook for a few minutes. Transfer beef in a bowl and keep it aside.
4. Rinse your cooking pan and heat two teaspoons oil again. Add carrots and mushroom and cook for three

minutes. It is time to add noodles and two tablespoons soy sauce blend. Cook for one minute and add only 1/3 cup water and cook to make noodles tender. It will take almost three minutes. Transfer noodles in a bowl with beef.

5. Clean skillet again and keep it on the heat again and add remaining sesame oil. Add remaining mixture of soy sauce and spinach and cook them for one minute. It is time to add beef and mix them well.

Nutritional Value per Serving:

- 450 Calories
- 12 grams of Fat
- 48 grams of Carbohydrates
- 37 grams of Protein

Benefits of this Recipe:

Beef

Beef contains a good amount of protein because it is mainly composed of it. With protein in beef, the breakdown of it is amino acids. Amino acids are crucial to health. It is similar to that of muscles in our body. In other words, protein is crucial to tissue building. Besides protein, beef contains a good number of vitamins and minerals.

Dinner Meal: Turkey Meatballs stuffed with Cheese

Think crispy on the outside, cheesy on the inside. That is what turkey meatballs stuffed with cheese can give you. This recipe is to die for, not literally.

Serving(s): 4-6

You will need:

- 1 lb. turkey meat, ground
- ½ cup mozzarella cheese, cut into bite sized cubes
- ½ cup grated Romano cheese
- 1 egg
- 5 garlic clove, minced
- 2 teaspoons fresh parsley, chopped
- 1 cup whole wheat panko bread
- ½ cup warm water
- 6 tablespoons olive oil
- 3 teaspoons Italian seasoning
- ½ teaspoon sugar
- 1 teaspoon salt
- ½ teaspoon red pepper flakes, crushed
- 1 can tomatoes, crushed
- 2 pinch of salt
- 1 pinch of pepper
- Salt and black pepper to taste

What to do:

1. Mix the turkey meat, egg, cheese, seasoning, parsley, half of the minced garlic, panko bread, salt and pepper. Mix well until you can shape it into meatballs

2. Preheat oven at 200 degrees Celsius.
3. Prepare a skillet over medium heat and add olive oil.
4. Use a tablespoon to scoop a piece of meat onto a baking sheet, place the cheese on top and cover it with another piece of meat. Roll the meat into meatballs.
5. Add the meatballs into your skillet to fry them. Fry the meatballs on all sides for about 1-2 minutes.
6. Take the meatballs out and place them back on the baking sheet to be baked in the oven for 10-12 minutes.
7. Add oil to your skillet pan over medium heat.
8. Add remaining garlic to be sautéed till golden.
9. Add the remaining ingredients (seasoning, pepper flakes, sugar, tomatoes, salt and pepper) to create your sauce. Simmer the mix for about 8 minutes. Add salt and pepper to taste.
10. By this time, your meatballs are ready to be added into the sauce mix.

Nutritional Value per Serving:

- 420 Calories
- 12 grams of Fat
- 19 grams of Carbohydrates
- 55 grams of Protein

Benefits of this Recipe:

Turkey Meat

The benefits of having turkey are:

- Great source of protein, iron, zinc, and potassium

- Lower cholesterol levels
- Low in fat
- Rich in Vitamin B6 and niacin for energy production
- Boosts immunity

Dinner Meal: Steak and Scramble Eggs

Whether it is for a breakfast or dinner, you can really enjoy the combination of steak and eggs.

Serving(s): 2

You will need:

- ½ cup lean sirloin steaks, cut into bite sized cubes
- 2 free range eggs
- 4 egg whites
- 2 teaspoons olive oil
- 1 medium potato, cut into bite sized cubes
- 1 teaspoon skim milk
- ¼ cup mushrooms
- 2 teaspoons Worcestershire sauce
- 2 tablespoons low-fat cheese, shredded
- 30 ml onions, chopped
- Paprika to taste
- Salt and black pepper to taste

What to do:

1. Heat a skillet pan over a medium-high heat.
2. Add oil, potatoes, onions, paprika and cook for 5 minutes. You may add salt and pepper to taste.
3. In a separate bowl, beat the eggs. Add milk as you continue to beat the egg.
4. Now, coming back to your pan, add Worcestershire sauce, mushrooms and the main dish, steak. Cook for about 4-6 minutes.
5. There will be excess fat from the pan mix. Drain the excess fat.
6. Add the eggs mix to the pan and scramble them together for about 4 minutes.

7. Once again, the dish is ready to serve. Sprinkle cheese to the dish and watch it melt just right.

Nutritional Value per Serving:

- 256 Calories
- 13 grams of Fat
- 22.8 grams of Carbohydrates
- 18.2 grams of Protein

Benefits of this Recipe:

Sirloin Steak

Sirloin steak is one of the healthiest cut of red meat. It is a lean cut of beef. Sirloin is located on the upper side of a cow. You can either grill, broil or sauté the sirloin. With this nutritious part of the beef, you can bet that you are getting a great addition to your diet plan. Benefits of sirloin steak are:

- Moderate amount of fat
- Great source of protein, iron, zinc, and vitamin B
- Macronutrients helpful for muscle growth and immunity boost

A great end to your meals and a ready to eat snack are these Amaretti Cookies. Each bite is soft and full of almond, fruity flavor. This recipe uses strawberry jam, but you can feel free to use any other sugar-free jams, which can be any flavor of your choice. A brand that you can look for is Polaner (it is the lowest option that you can use).

Serving(s): 16

You will need:

- 1 cup of Almond Flour
- 1 tablespoon of Coconut Flour
- ½ teaspoon of Baking Powder
- ¼ teaspoon of Cinnamon
- ½ teaspoon of Salt
- ½ cup of Erythritol (*Natural Sweetener*)
- 2 large Eggs
- 4 tablespoon of Coconut Oil
- ½ teaspoon Vanilla Extract
- ½ teaspoon Almond Extract
- 2 tablespoon Sugar-Free Jam
- 1 tablespoon Organic Shredded Coconut (*Shredded Coconut*)

What to do:

1. Pre-heat your oven to 350 Fahrenheit. While you're at it, combine all your dry ingredients and whisk it around. Make sure it is properly mixed.
2. Add in your wet ingredients into your mixing bowl and whisk it.
3. Prepare a parchment paper on top of a tray and line the baking sheet with it. Form your cookies on the tray

and make a small indent circle in the middle of the cookie, while using your finger or you can use the back of a teaspoon.

4. Bake it for 16 minutes or until it looks golden, cooked and slightly cracked.
5. Cool the cookies on a wire rack for around 10 minutes and place your jam on top of the cookie.
6. Sprinkle with the coconut on top of each cookie and get ready to snack it out or if you want to keep it stored to be prepared for your next dessert.

Nutritional Value per Serving:

- 86 Calories
- 7.9 grams of Fats
- 1.2 grams of Net Carbohydrate
- 2.4 grams of Protein

Benefits of this Recipe:

Cinnamon

Who can't resist this highly delicious spice? Other than being such a great combination with food, it has also been prized for medicinal purposes throughout the years:

- Highly potent antioxidants, which have anti-inflammatory effects
- Improves heart disease, including cholesterol, triglycerides and blood pressure
- Reduce blood sugar levels

Coconut Oil

Once again, coconut is a great source of benefits for your body. The oil is not just used in the tropical countries, where coconut is abundant, but, also in the UK and US. As people discover more about coconut, they realize all the wonders and benefits it can produce.

- Great skin care for fighting dry skin
- Beneficial for those with heart disease
- Useful for weight loss
- Strengthens immune system

Snack: Raspberry Lemon Popsicles

(Great to beat the summer heat)

These popsicles can be stored in a freezer and kept for when you need to cool down from the heat of the sun. Usual Ketogenic popsicles are hard and have a grainier texture, but this recipe is guaranteed smooth and creamy.

Serving(s): 6

You will need:

- Immersion Blender (Helps to blend the mixture smoothly)
- 100 grams of Raspberries
- ½ Lemon Juice
- ¼ Cup of Coconut Oil
- 1 Cup of Coconut Milk (Carton)
- ¼ Cup of Sour Cream
- ¼ Cup of Heavy Cream
- ½ teaspoon of Guar Gum
- 20 drops of Liquid Stevia

What to do:

1. Add all the ingredients into a container and make sure you use an immersion blender to blend the mixture together
2. Continue blending and add the raspberries into the mixture and mix until smooth
3. Strain the mixture and throw away any leftover raspberry seeds.
4. Pour the mixture into the mold you want and set the popsicles in the freezer overnight or for a minimum time of 2 hours

5. Once frozen, run the mold under hot water ad dislodge the popsicles
6. Serve when you want or store in the fridge for a great snack!

Nutritional Value per Serving:

- 151 Calories
- 16 grams of Fats
- 2 grams of Carbohydrates
- 0.5 grams of Protein

Snack: Crispy Catfish

Serving(s): 2

You will need:

- ½ cup buttermilk
- 1 ½ cups fine cornmeal
- ½ cup all-purpose flour
- ½ cup water
- 1 teaspoon seafood seasoning
- Pepper and salt as per taste
- 1-quart vegetable oil
- 1 pound Catfish fillets (strips)

What to do:

1. Take one small bowl and mix water, salt, pepper, and buttermilk. Pour this mixture into a flat pan (large enough to handle fish fillets). Spread fish fillets on this spread and turn well to coat each side. Keep them aside to marinate.
2. Take a plastic bag and add seafood seasoning, flour and cornmeal. Mix them well and add fish fillets in this mixture. Put a few fillets at one time and gently coat them equally.
3. Take a deep fryer and heat oil at 365 degrees F and deep fry all fish fillets to make them golden brown. It will take almost 3 minutes. Make sure to fry fish fillets in small batches to make each fillet crispy and golden brown. Drain these fillets on plates lined with paper towels. Serve with your favorite dip or sauce.

Nutritional Value per Serving:

- 155 Calories
- 8 grams of Fats
- 1.2 grams of Carbohydrates
- 14 grams of Protein

This is plain, simple and easy to make. You can use this to put over some of that Cauliflower rice mentioned above.

Serving(s): 4

You will need:

- 4 ounces of Breakfast Sausage
- 2 tablespoon of Butter
- 1 Cup of Heavy Cream
- ½ teaspoon of Guar Gum
- Salt and Pepper to taste

What to do:

1. Place sausage into the pan and make sure that it browns well.
2. Remove the sausage from the pan and make sure the fat is still kept there. Add 2-tablespoon butter onto the pan and let it melt.
3. Once the butter has been completely melted, add the heavy cream and stir it until it boils
4. Add the guar gum to make it thicker and stir until boiled. Let the mixture thicken and run the spatula through it, if it takes a moment to close the gap on the pan, then it's ready.
5. Add sausage back into the pan and stir!

Nutritional Value per Serving:

- 346 Calories
- 38 grams of Fat
- 1.5 grams of Net Carbohydrates

- 4 grams of Protein

Breakfast Sausage

Whether you believe it or not, breakfast sausages can provide you with some benefit too!

- Protein
- Vitamins B12
- Iron

Guar Gum

This is a food additive and a natural food thickener. In this recipe it is used to thicken the gravy

- Lowers blood cholesterol
- Slows rate of starch digestion and glucose absorption
- Lowers possibility of diarrhea

Serving(s): 2

You will need:

- 2 tablespoons of Peanut Butter or Nut Butter, just make sure that whatever it is made out of is just nuts and salt
- ½ cup of Coconut Cream
- 1 cup of Milk (Suggested: Almond, Whole Milk, Heavy Cream)
- 1 teaspoon of Vanilla Extract
- 1 cup of Ice
- Stevia (To taste or 1/8 would be great)

What to do:

1. Just blend it all together and place it in a nice mason jar and you've got a delicious cup of healthy and nutritious Ketogenic Peanut Butter Milkshake!

Benefits of this Recipe:

Nut Butter

Spreadable foodstuff usually made from grinding nuts into a paste and it is super delicious when placed with some bread.

- High in protein
- Healthy Fats
- Abundance of fiber
- Phytochemicals (Which actually, helps prevent cancer, according to American Cancer Society)

Coconut Cream

Similar to coconut milk, but it contains less amount of water. The main difference between the two is its consistency with each other.

- Improves immunity
- Gives energy, not fat
- Slows down aging (especially when this ingredient is placed in a face cream)
- Hydrates your body

You have now been blessed with recipes that are sure to satisfy your taste buds while giving you great health benefits with deliciousness! It helps to just try out a recipe or two first to get yourself started.

Part IV – Time to Burn Those Fat

The Ketogenic Diet focuses on losing fat in the body by adjusting our diet. Exercise is also a great way to lose fat stimulating your metabolism to burn more fat. There are two types of exercises that a person can perform to burn fat and speed up their metabolism. The first being High-Intensity Interval Training and the second is Weightlifting. We will discuss the physiology behind each one in regards to losing fat and different routines and exercises you can perform. Let us begin with High-Intensity Interval Training.

High-Intensity Interval Training (HIIT)

This is the type of workout is abbreviated as HIIT and they are composed of a short burst of intense movements and exercises that get the heart pumping, your fat burning and a person very exhausted. These include sprints, short intense swims, and heavy weight lifting. This is the opposite of Low-Intensity Interval Training (abbreviated as LIIT) which are long walks or jogs, riding a bike at low speed or lifting light weights.

Keep in mind that what might be LIIT for one person can be considered a very difficult HIIT exercise for another. A trained athlete can train much harder and longer than a person who has very little to no training, is getting back into training or is overweight. An example would be a person with weak muscles walking up a hill for 2 minutes which to them feels like an HIIT exercise while for a trained athlete this might not be considered a workout at all. We must keep everything in perspective and adjust accordingly. For the purposes of this book, we'll consider you the reader, as a non-trained aspiring fitness lover who is going to start from scratch.

One easy and fun way to view HIIT is you playing a sport such as basketball or football. Sports that involve a quick burst of intense movement followed by a short rest period (stop and start) are HIIT by nature.

When we do HIIT we are looking to get a hormonal response that will cause shifts in our metabolism which will result in a loss of fat. With that said, your tenth day of HIIT training will be 100 times harder than your first. This is because if we do not continually increase the difficulty of our training then we will not get a hormonal response.

If you really want to start from scratch and get a full experience of what HIIT feels like, then put on some running shoes and try this fundamental HIIT workout. If you have access to a running track (it's called a Tartan Track for those of you wondering) then much better. You are simply going to sprint on the straightaways on the track and lightly jog or even walk on the curves, this is what you call "Ins and Outs." If you do not have access to a track, then you can take this workout to the roads. You can simply sprint for one block and walk the next. First, you are going start easy with maybe 2 - 3 laps and then increase by one lap every time you do the workout. This is HIIT at its most basic form and is a sure fat burner.

It is highly recommended that you participate in sports that involve HIIT since you will have a lot more fun and as an end result you will get more work done. Remember, the more intense your workout the greater hormonal response you will get. Therefore, the more work you put in the better your results.

Now let us talk about weightlifting and its benefits to fat loss.

The stereotype of getting into shape is walking into a gym and curling a dumbbell for an hour and then leaving, which is true up to the part where you walk into the gym. The time you spend in the gym is not long and the exercises you choose to do are very important. The reason HIIT training is so effective is because it incorporates the whole body in an intense movement and workout. This same concept applies to weightlifting; you want to do exercises that incorporate as many muscles in one movement as possible. These types of exercises are called Compound Exercises and there are 4 main movements. A vertical push, horizontal push, vertical pull, and a horizontal pull.

This means that we can walk into the gym and get a killer workout that will stimulate our hormones and metabolism in a quick (notice how I didn't say easy) four workouts. Let us begin with the vertical push compound exercise and the king of all fat burners, The Squat.

Squatting is the king of all workouts because of every of the muscle group is needed to lift the weight. You will position yourself under the bar, place the bar along your upper back and then squat all the way down.

As for weight, start very low to get a feel of what having a weight on your body feels like and then slowly move up. I recommend starting with just 10lbs on each side for you first try. You will come to see that the Squat is one of the most very demanding exercises out there so you should begin your workout with The Squat. Do four sets at 6 - 8 repetitions per set and you will be losing fat in no time.

For our second workout, we are going to be looking at the Bench Press which brings our chest, shoulder, triceps and core (belly) into one fun workout. You are just going to lay flat on your back under a bar, lift it from the rack, lower the bar to your chest and repeat. Start on a low weight so you can get used to the movement and do same sets/repetitions as the Squats.

For our third exercise, we will be doing a Deadlift. This workout is the opposite of a Squat where instead of putting a weight above our head and squatting down, we will instead put a weight on the floor and pull it up. This is an amazing full body workout that stimulates the metabolism and generates hormonal responses since we are using almost every muscle in our body to lift the weight. As for set and repetitions, I recommend 3 sets of 5 repetitions.

For our last workout, you are going to do a Row. Almost every gym has the Row machine where you will sit on the machine, grab the handles and pull back (as if you are rowing a boat.) This is a full back workout and not as difficult as the other three. Do the same number of sets and repetitions as the Squat.

Out of these four exercises that we went over, the most important one is The Squat. If you are short on time or not very much of a gym goer, then you can simply just do Squats. Make sure the weight is a little heavier and do six sets and 6 - 9 repetitions each. Remember, the point of working out is the generate a hormonal response that speeds up your metabolism that will result in burning a lot of calories.

Part V – How to End the Ketogenic Diet

There are a number of reasons of why a person may want to end this awesome diet. One of them being that a person has already met their goal in terms of weight and fitness and no longer wish to continue. Others love eating and find that the fun is taken of the experience when we have to count calories, macros and watch what we eat. Lastly, some due to their demographics do not have access to the foods needed for the Keto Diet to succeed. Now there are a lot of symptoms that come along with the diet early on, so it's best to try and stick to the diet for at least four weeks before truly deciding that this diet was not meant for you. It's important to understand that those "terrible" feelings are all part of the journey and is just something you have to go through when starting the ketogenic diet.

The trick to stopping a keto diet is graduation or in other words, achieving the goals you have set for yourself. Once a person decides to reintroduce carbs back into his life, he has to build his carb intake slowly and steadily, not rapidly. This means gradually adding carbs little by little each day. One way someone can do this is by adding ten grams of carbs each day. If any problems surface, simply add less than ten grams a day and just try to feel out what works for you. It's also important to understand that "gaining" weight after stopping the diet is unavoidable. Most people gain about 5 pounds of water weight when ending their diet. What happens is that your body will build back its reserves of glycogen due to the reintroduction of carbs. That glycogen will store water, which is the main reason that accounts for the increase in weight.

There are a lot of horror stories out there that talk about how people who stopped their ketogenic diets gained everything back. This is a common myth. As explained before, you will gain water weight, but unless you go back to the way you were eating which made you put on that extra weight in the first place, you should be fine. After ending the diet, it's important to remain health conscious. For most people who were on the diet, remaining health conscious should not at all be difficult because they had to be health conscious during the diet. The key to any diet is that you cannot truly go back to your old habits.

The ketogenic diet doesn't just make people lose weight. It also teaches them how to refine the way they look at food. It even has helped out with some people's cooking ability and overall confidence. Just remember that the symptoms you experience early on in the keto diet are only temporary. It's all part of adapting. Try to stick with the diet for a month and if you really aren't enjoying the benefits, maybe it's time to move on to something else.

Part VI – Conclusion

Thank you again for purchasing this book!

The Ketogenic Diet has been a great aid to people who having been trying to lose weight and burn fat. We have gone over different recipes you can try so that you won't feel bored or limited on the diet. The combination of a high protein and good fat diet with low carbs are key to this diet. The overall goal is to improve your blood sugar, cholesterol and get our bodies to use our fats for energy.

In may take some time to get used to having low carbs in your diet but once you get the hang of it, you'll starting feeling good and looking even better. Remember that you can add exercises to with your diet even better results and that there will come a time where this awesome diet must end.

Once you end the diet, do not go back to your old eating habits. This is a journey that you will embark on to better your life and once it reaches an end you realize that it will have resonating effects on your life that will change you forever. I wish you luck on your journey and a healthy life.

Finally, if you have enjoyed reading this book and have benefited from it, I'd like to ask a favor if you could be kind enough to leave a review for this book on Amazon? Much appreciated.

Thank you!

Strawberry Cheesecake Fat Bombs

Ingredients:

- ½ cup of fresh or frozen strawberries
- ¾ cup of softened cream cheese
- ¼ cup of softened butter or coconut oil
- 2 tablespoons of powdered erythritol (*Or 10 – 15 drops of liquid stevia*)
- 1 vanilla bean (*Or ½ - 1 tablespoon of vanilla extract*)

Instructions:

1. Cut the softened butter in smaller pieces.
2. Place the cream cheese and cut butter into a mixing bowl and leave it at room temperature for about 30 – 60 minutes until it becomes softened.
3. Wash the strawberries and remove the leaves.
4. Place them into a bowl and start mashing them up with a fork or you can also choose to place them in a blender to smoothen the texture.
5. Add powered erythritol, vanilla extract and mix them well together.
6. Before you mix the strawberries with the other ingredients, make sure it is in room temperature.
7. Add to the bowl with softened butter and cream cheese.
8. Use a whisk or food processor in order to mix it well together.
9. Spoon the mixture into small silicone muffin molds or a candy mold of your choice.
10. Place in the freezer to let it set for about 2 hours.
11. Once done, unmold the fat bombs and place in a container for storage.

Check out the rest of *Ketogenic Fat Bomb Recipes* on Amazon.

Check out my other books

I'd like to share my other books. Simply search for my books on Amazon.

Ketogenic Fat Bomb Recipes by Caitlin Johansson

Ketogenic Diet: 7-Day Ketogenic Diet Plan & Recipes for Rapid Weight Loss by Caitlin Johansson

CPSIA information can be obtained
at www.ICGtesting.com
Printed in the USA
LVOW13s0426110517
534081LV00012B/603/P